FREEDOM
FROM
PNUEMONIA

DIVINE MEDICINE THAT WORKS

BY
IHEKE WILLIAMS

Unless otherwise indicated, all scripture quotations are taken from the King James Version of the Bible. A key for other Bible versions used;

NKJV	New King James Version
AMP	The Amplified Bible
TANT	The New Amplified Bible
TLB -	The Living Bible
CEV -	Contemporary English Version
NASB	New American Standard Version
GW -	God's Word version
ESV -	English Standard Version
NET -	New English Translation
ISV -	International Standard Version
NIV -	New International Version
MSG -	The Message Translation

<u>DEDICATION</u>

This Book is dedicated to Almighty God
and to everyone in the world.

TABLE OF CONTENT

WHAT IS PNUEMONIA?

Pneumonia is an inflammatory condition of the lung affecting primarily the small air sacs known as alveoli. Typically symptoms include some combination of productive or dry cough, chest pain, fever and trouble breathing. Severity is variable

Source: Wikipedia

WHAT IS GOD'S SOLUTION

But He was wounded for our transgressions, he was bruised for our iniquities: the chastisement of our peace was upon Him; and with His stripes we are healed – Isaiah 53:5 (KJV)

"...By His wounds ye have been healed" – 1 Peter 2:24 (KJV)

The phrase "...ye <u>HAVE BEEN HEALED</u>" is in the past tense, it means JESUS has ALREADY HEALED you from pneumonia over 2000 years ago.

You have NO business with Pneumonia.

The air sacs of your lungs are Healed already, free and active Forever because of the sufferings of Christ on the cross for your sake.

For the next 31 days and forever, you will affirm this blessing that Our Lord Jesus Christ has given to you and you will you live in perfect health FOREVER!.

INSTRUCTION 1

That if thou shalt <u>confess with thy mouth</u> the Lord Jesus, and shalt <u>believe in thine heart</u> that God hath raised him from the dead, thou shalt be saved. – Romans 10:9

We having the same <u>spirit of faith</u>, according as it is written, I believed, and therefore have I spoken; <u>we also believe, and therefore speak</u>; - 2 Corinthians 4:13

There has to be a connection with what you say/affirm with your mouth and what you have in your heart or what you believe in your heart.

Consequently, for the affirmations to be effective, you will have to meditate on the scripture (1 Peter 2:24) for 5 minutes, in your heart, before you affirm it with your mouth.

Don't say anything to the contrary during the period of affirmations.

INSTRUCTION 2

"For our light affliction, which is but for a moment, worketh for us a far more exceeding and eternal weight of glory;

While we look not at the things which are seen, but at the things which are not seen: for the things which are seen are temporal; but the things which are not seen are eternal. – 2 Corinthians 4:17-18 (KJV)

For the duration of the affirmations, do not touch any part of your body that might have been affected by this sickness. If it is possible, don't look at it.

The word of God (1 Peter 2:24) in your heart will <u>not</u> be effective when you keep recognizing the presence of a sickness because doubt will begin to develop in your heart and the word doesn't work in the presence of doubts/unbelief.

Follow these instructions, **BE CONSISTENT** and your affirmations will be very effective.

DAY 1
AFFIRMATION

Meditate on 1 Peter 2:24B
in your heart for 5 minutes

"..By His stripes ye have
been healed"

NOW say the words below to
yourself

"I HAVE BEEN HEALED
THEREFORE, I AFFIRM
THAT I DO NOT HAVE
PNEUMONIA !"

DAY 2
AFFIRMATION

Meditate on 1 Peter 2:24B
in your heart for 5 minutes

"..By His stripes ye have
been healed"

NOW say the words below to
yourself

"I HAVE BEEN HEALED
THEREFORE, I AFFIRM
THAT MY BODY IS
ACTIVE AND STRONG
FOREVER!"

DAY 3
AFFIRMATION

Meditate on 1 Peter 2:24B
in your heart for 5 minutes

"..By His stripes ye have
been healed"

NOW say the words below to
yourself

**"I HAVE BEEN HEALED
THEREFORE, I AFFIRM
THAT MY LUNG IS FREE
AND ACTIVE!"**

DAY 4
AFFIRMATION

Meditate on 1 Peter 2:24B
in your heart for 5 minutes

"..By His stripes ye have
been healed"

NOW say the words below to yourself

"I HAVE BEEN HEALED THEREFORE, I AFFIRM THAT I DO NOT HAVE PNEUMONIA !"

DAY 5
AFFIRMATION

Meditate on 1 Peter 2:24B
in your heart for 5 minutes

"..By His stripes ye have
been healed"

NOW say the words below to
yourself

"I HAVE BEEN HEALED
THEREFORE, I AFFIRM
THAT MY LUNG IS FREE
AND ACTIVE!"

DAY 6
AFFIRMATION

Meditate on 1 Peter 2:24B
in your heart for 5 minutes

"..By His stripes ye have
been healed"

NOW say the words below to
yourself

"I HAVE BEEN HEALED
THEREFORE, I AFFIRM
THAT I DO NOT HAVE
PNEUMONIA !"

DAY 7
AFFIRMATION

Meditate on 1 Peter 2:24B
in your heart for 5 minutes

"..By His stripes ye have
been healed"

NOW say the words below to
yourself

"I HAVE BEEN HEALED
THEREFORE, I AFFIRM
THAT MY LUNG IS FREE
AND ACTIVE!"

DAY 8
AFFIRMATION

Meditate on 1 Peter 2:24B
in your heart for 5 minutes

"..By His stripes ye have
been healed"

NOW say the words below to
yourself

"I HAVE BEEN HEALED
THEREFORE, I AFFIRM
THAT I DO NOT HAVE
PNEUMONIA !"

DAY 9
AFFIRMATION

Meditate on 1 Peter 2:24B
in your heart for 5 minutes

"..By His stripes ye have
been healed"

NOW say the words below to
yourself

"I HAVE BEEN HEALED THEREFORE, I AFFIRM THAT MY LUNG IS FREE AND ACTIVE!"

DAY 10
AFFIRMATION

Meditate on 1 Peter 2:24B
in your heart for 5 minutes

"..By His stripes ye have
been healed"

NOW say the words below to
yourself

"I HAVE BEEN HEALED THEREFORE, I AFFIRM THAT I DO NOT HAVE PNEUMONIA !"

DAY 11
AFFIRMATION

Meditate on 1 Peter 2:24B
in your heart for 5 minutes

"..By His stripes ye have
been healed"

NOW say the words below to
yourself

"I HAVE BEEN HEALED
THEREFORE, I AFFIRM
THAT MY LUNG IS FREE
AND ACTIVE!"

DAY 12
AFFIRMATION

Meditate on 1 Peter 2:24B
in your heart for 5 minutes

"..By His stripes ye have
been healed"

NOW say the words below to
yourself

"I HAVE BEEN HEALED
THEREFORE, I AFFIRM
THAT I DO NOT HAVE
PNEUMONIA !"

DAY 13
AFFIRMATION

Meditate on 1 Peter 2:24B
in your heart for 5 minutes

"..By His stripes ye have
been healed"

NOW say the words below to
yourself

"I HAVE BEEN HEALED
THEREFORE, I AFFIRM
THAT MY LUNG IS FREE
AND ACTIVE!"

DAY 14
AFFIRMATION

Meditate on 1 Peter 2:24B
in your heart for 5 minutes

"..By His stripes ye have
been healed"

NOW say the words below to
yourself

"I HAVE BEEN HEALED
THEREFORE, I AFFIRM
THAT I DO NOT HAVE
PNEUMONIA !"

DAY 15
AFFIRMATION

Meditate on 1 Peter 2:24B
in your heart for 5 minutes

"..By His stripes ye have
been healed"

NOW say the words below to
yourself

"I HAVE BEEN HEALED
THEREFORE, I AFFIRM
THAT MY LUNG IS
FREE AND ACTIVE!"

DAY 16
AFFIRMATION

Meditate on 1 Peter 2:24B
in your heart for 5 minutes

" ..By His stripes ye have
been healed"

NOW say the words below to
yourself

"I HAVE BEEN HEALED
THEREFORE, I AFFIRM
THAT I DO NOT HAVE
PNEUMONIA !"

DAY 17
AFFIRMATION

Meditate on 1 Peter 2:24B
in your heart for 5 minutes

"..By His stripes ye have
been healed"

NOW say the words below to
yourself

"I HAVE BEEN HEALED
THEREFORE, I AFFIRM
THAT MY LUNG IS
FREE AND ACTIVE!"

DAY 18
AFFIRMATION

Meditate on 1 Peter 2:24B
in your heart for 5 minutes

"..By His stripes ye have
been healed"

NOW say the words below to
yourself

"I HAVE BEEN HEALED
THEREFORE, I AFFIRM
THAT I DO NOT HAVE
PNEUMONIA !"

DAY 19
AFFIRMATION

Meditate on 1 Peter 2:24B
in your heart for 5 minutes

"..By His stripes ye have
been healed"

NOW say the words below to
yourself

"I HAVE BEEN HEALED
THEREFORE, I AFFIRM
THAT MY LUNG IS
FREE AND ACTIVE!"

DAY 20
AFFIRMATION

Meditate on 1 Peter 2:24B
in your heart for 5 minutes

"..By His stripes ye have
been healed"

NOW say the words below to
yourself

"I HAVE BEEN HEALED
THEREFORE, I AFFIRM
THAT I DO NOT HAVE
PNEUMONIA !"

DAY 21
AFFIRMATION

Meditate on 1 Peter 2:24B
in your heart for 5 minutes

" ..By His stripes ye have
been healed"

NOW say the words below to
yourself

"I HAVE BEEN HEALED
THEREFORE, I AFFIRM
THAT MY LUNG IS
FREE AND ACTIVE!"

DAY 22
AFFIRMATION

Meditate on 1 Peter 2:24B
in your heart for 5 minutes

"..By His stripes ye have
      been healed"

NOW say the words below to
yourself

"I HAVE BEEN HEALED
THEREFORE, I AFFIRM
THAT I DO NOT HAVE
PNEUMONIA !"

DAY 23
AFFIRMATION

Meditate on 1 Peter 2:24B
in your heart for 5 minutes

"..By His stripes ye have
been healed"

NOW say the words below to
yourself

"I HAVE BEEN HEALED THEREFORE, I AFFIRM THAT MY LUNG IS FREE AND ACTIVE!"

DAY 24
AFFIRMATION

Meditate on 1 Peter 2:24B
in your heart for 5 minutes

"..By His stripes ye have
been healed"

NOW say the words below to
yourself

"I HAVE BEEN HEALED
THEREFORE, I AFFIRM
THAT I DO NOT HAVE
PNEUMONIA !"

DAY 25
AFFIRMATION

Meditate on 1 Peter 2:24B
in your heart for 5 minutes

"..By His stripes ye have
been healed"

NOW say the words below to
yourself

"I HAVE BEEN HEALED
THEREFORE, I AFFIRM
THAT MY LUNG IS
FREE AND ACTIVE!"

DAY 26
AFFIRMATION

Meditate on 1 Peter 2:24B
in your heart for 5 minutes

" ..By His stripes ye have
been healed"

NOW say the words below to
yourself

"I HAVE BEEN HEALED
THEREFORE, I AFFIRM
THAT I DO NOT HAVE
PNEUMONIA !"

DAY 27
AFFIRMATION

Meditate on 1 Peter 2:24B
in your heart for 5 minutes

"..By His stripes ye have
been healed"

NOW say the words below to
yourself

"I HAVE BEEN HEALED
THEREFORE, I AFFIRM
THAT THE AIR SACS OF
MY LUNGS ARE FREE,
ACTIVE AND PERFECT!"

DAY 28
AFFIRMATION

Meditate on 1 Peter 2:24B
in your heart for 5 minutes

" ..By His stripes ye have
been healed"

NOW say the words below to
yourself

"I HAVE BEEN HEALED
THEREFORE, I AFFIRM
THAT I DO NOT HAVE
PNEUMONIA !"

DAY 29
AFFIRMATION

Meditate on 1 Peter 2:24B
in your heart for 5 minutes

"..By His stripes ye have
been healed"

NOW say the words below to
yourself

"I HAVE BEEN HEALED
THEREFORE, I AFFIRM
THAT MY LUNG IS
FREE AND ACTIVE!"

DAY 30
AFFIRMATION

Meditate on 1 Peter 2:24B
in your heart for 5 minutes

"..By His stripes ye have
been healed"

NOW say the words below to
yourself

"I HAVE BEEN HEALED
THEREFORE, I AFFIRM
THAT I DO NOT HAVE
PNEUMONIA !"

DAY 31
AFFIRMATION

Meditate on 1 Peter 2:24B
in your heart for 5 minutes

"..By His stripes ye have
been healed"

NOW say the words below to
yourself

"I HAVE BEEN HEALED THEREFORE, I AFFIRM THAT MY LUNG IS FREE AND ACTIVE!"

"..by His stripes ye
HAVE BEEN HEALED"-
1 PETER 2:24

Jesus Christ has paid the price for your peace. Don't let Satan deceive you that you are sick.

Don't let Satan put you in bondage any longer.

Your body has been healed already. You have NO business with sickness.

You are ACTIVE AND STRONG FOREVER!

You are FREE from pneumonia FOREVER!

PRAYER FOR SALVATION

We believe that you have been blessed and that you want to receive eternal life that God has made available to everyone who believes in his love and his grace which He expressed lavishly through His Son Jesus Christ.

"For God so loved the world, that He gave his only begotten Son, that whosoever _believeth_ in him should not perish, but _have everlasting life._" - John 3:16

Say this prayer to God and believe it with your heart

"Father, I believe that you gave me your only Son to die for my sin. I believe you raised Him from the dead. I declare that your son, Jesus Christ is the Lord of my life. I receive eternal life and I receive the Holy Spirit. I am saved forever.in Jesus name. I am so Happy that today and forever, I am your child. Amen ".

Congratulations, you are now a child of God Halleluyah!! – John 1:12

OTHER INFORMATION

Please share your testimonies via the following handles;

ihekewilliams@gmail.com
+2348061530541

Other Books written by the author includes

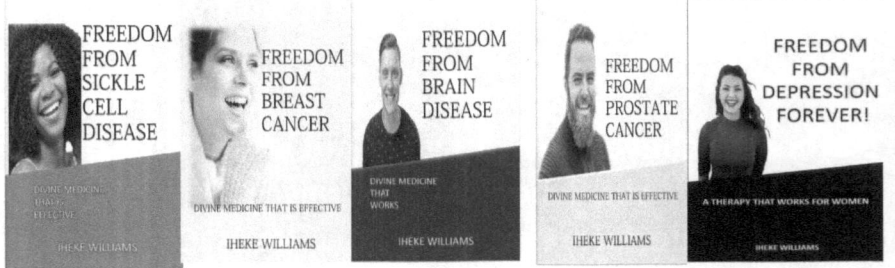

Visit us on Amazon by clicking on the link below;

https://www.amazon.com/Iheke-w.-Okpara/e/B01KFYO1PU/ref=ntt_dp_epwbk_0

ABOUT THE AUTHOR

Iheke Williams is a firm follower and disciple of the Lord Jesus Christ. He is a passionate minister of the grace of our Lord and savior Jesus Christ and has brought the reality of the divine life of Christ into the lives of so many.

Iheke Williams has a calling to communicate the gospel of Christ with simplicity and to show the world how to activate the eternal life of God that is in us already which includes Divine health, Divine righteousness, Divine security and Divine prosperity.

As you read this book and other books written by Iheke Williams you will literally begin to function and manifest the life of God that is already inside you to the glory of God the Father who is the author of all grace and mercy. Amen.

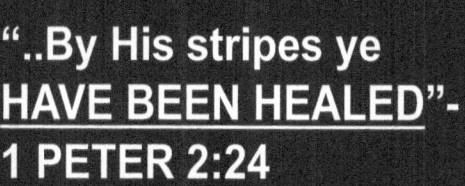

"..By His stripes ye
HAVE BEEN HEALED"-
1 PETER 2:24

YOU
ARE
FREE
FOREVER!!

FREEDOM SERIES

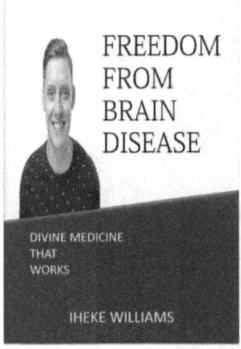

https://www.amazon.com/Iheke-w.-Okpara/e/B01KFYO1PU/ref=ntt_dp_epwbk_0

www.ingramcontent.com/pod-product-compliance
Lightning Source LLC
Chambersburg PA
CBHW061228280526
45784CB00006B/2682